Table of Contents

Introduction:

There are many reasons why people are getting into making their own homemade soaps: they may want to control the ingredients that are simple and natural, allergies to common big box soap ingredients, getting back to basics, or being more self-sufficient.

Now that we have that out of the way, let's get down to business! Why did I start making my own soap? I wanted to be in control of the ingredients, and as my website states "Getting Back to Basics" because I want to be more self-sufficient and self-reliant.

The first thing I did was buy all the necessary equipment that I did not have already and bought the ingredients needed to make the most basic soap: Castile Soap. To say the least, with all the information I read about lye and adding it to water, I was nervous! However, my first batch of soap was made without any complications and I have used it over the last few months.

All recommendations from this book are 100% natural, including scents and colorants. What is the point of making an "all-natural" soap homemade, if you put toxic ingredients into the finishing product to make it colorful?

I hope you are just excited to make soap as I was the first time!!

Chapter One: Understanding about Soap

In this chapter, I will explain the background on soap, benefits of making your own soap, and the basics of soap.

What Is Soap?

Soap is created during the chemical process called saponification when the lye water is added to the oils.

Soap has been around for centuries, dating as far back to around 2800 BC in ancient Babylon. The first "written" soap recipe dates back to 2200 BC on a Babylonian clay tablet that consisted of water, alkali, and cassia oil.

Farmers were known to use every part of the animal and would use the fat of the animal to make soap and even candles.

Benefits of Making Your Own Soap

Before delving into any project, the benefits of the project need to be understood. There are many great benefits to soap making.

- You control the ingredients – you know exactly what the product is made of. There are no artificial ingredients or ingredients that the government defines as "generally recognized as safe". Everything recommended, as stated before, will be 100% natural; no artificial fillers here! ☺

- You become more self-sufficient – as you learn the process of making soap, you will no longer rely on the "big box" stores to have soap. You can make your own.
- You want to save money – even though there will be some up-front costs in the initial starting of making your own soap, these costs can be minimal, and over time, will pay for itself.
- You will be proud – I know that I was after my first batch of soap. I was so happy and it worked! Which made me even more ecstatic about accomplishing this.

There are many benefits to making your own soap, but ultimately, you have to decide if this is something you want to do for yourself and your family.

Basics of Soap Making

The basics of soap making need to be understood before you can actually make soap. For saponification to occur, fatty acids and sodium hydroxide have to mix. The fatty acids are the butters, oils, and fats used in your recipes and sodium hydroxide is the lye that is used. Most recipes call for three or more oils because this gives the soap a great combination of benefits, including: cleansing, conditioning, moisturizing, acne reducer, and anti-aging.

The oils and fats used in soap making will be weighed and then added to a metal pot and melted together. After the oils and fats are melted, it will need to cool to 100° F - 110° F. As the oils and fats are melting, the water can be weighed in a glass bowl and in a separate bowl, measure the lye. Wearing your safety gear, which is covered in another section, slowly pour the lye into the water, mixing with a metal spoon. The mixture will then need to cool to 100° F - 110° F.

Once both the oils and fats and the lye/water mixture are both cooled, the lye/water will be added to the oils and fats and brought to trace. Trace is when the mixture just starts to show a trail across the mixture when you drizzle some over the top.

This is an example of soap brought to trace:

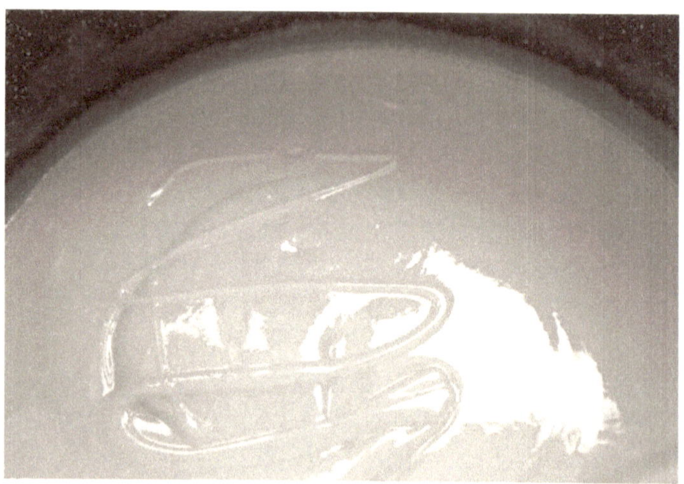

Once brought to trace, other additives can be added, such as essential oils and colorants. Then mixed again for a final few seconds and then the mixture is poured into the mold, insulated for at least 24 hours, then it can be cut and cured for 4 to 6 weeks.

Chapter Two:
Getting Your Supplies

In this chapter, I will explain all the supplies you will need.

There really isn't much equipment you need to start making soaps, however, the best option is to keep the equipment that is used for soap making separate from your standard kitchen equipment. Metal and/or glass is the best option in most cases also. There are many places you can also get some of the standard equipment for much less, such as thrift stores or garage sales.

Safety First!!

Safety Equipment will be the most important purchase and will need to be worn EVERYTIME you mix the lye into the water. Do NOT ever rush this process and always use caution. Do not ever feel you have this "mastered" and never had a problem so you do not need to wear anything this time. When lye is first mixed into water, the temperature becomes very hot, very quickly and can burn very easily. It also produces a fume that last about a minute, which can be toxic.

**Always mix your lye into the water, and do so outside to prevent the fumes being in the house and someone inhaling them
If used properly, however, there is nothing to be concerned about.

You will need to think about eye protection. Safety glasses or goggles is very important to have when working with lye. You want to ensure your eyes are protected from any splashing that may occur when pouring or mixing the lye into the water.

A safety mask is great to have to keep you from smelling the fumes when the lye is mixed into the water. Make sure the mask covers your mouth and nose and there are reusable ones available at most any store, including Amazon.

You will also want to wear gloves. Standard kitchen gloves that are used to wash dishes or clean the stove work well, even though they are bulky. Disposable gloves are just as good and not as bulky. This is more personal preference.

Clothes that protect your skin should be worn also. Long sleeves and long pants that cover all exposed skin is recommended for the same reason as wearing safety glasses or goggles; splashing could cause burns as the lye, once mixed in with the water, becomes very hot, very fast. Lye can also bleach fabric, so make sure the clothes you choose to wear, you do not mind getting ruined (if this happens).

Needed Equipment:

Most equipment needed can probably be found around the kitchen, however, there may be a few things that need to be purchased. Always keep your soap making equipment separate from your food equipment. Although it is soap, it contains raw lye which you definitely do not want to ingest.

A large stainless steel point will be necessary to melt the oils and then pour the lye/water mixture into. It needs to be large enough so there will be no chance of any splashing.

A digital scale and digital thermometer are excellent to have also. You can go with non-digital, but for the scale, you will need to ensure it can read in ounces as this is the standard for weighing the ingredients of the soap.

A stick blender makes the process of blending the lye/water mixture into the oils much easier; it isn't absolutely necessary, but you will spend a great deal of time mixing if doing it manually. There are some fairly cheap ones out there and I have a link to one on Amazon on my blog.

Molds are necessary to pouring the soap into so it will cure and be in blocks. You can purchase these, such as the one I recommend on Amazon, but many standard household items can be used also. Just keep in mind, some household items will require parchment paper inside the mold to prevent the soap from sticking and they might not be reusable, such as a cardboard box. There are many different types of molds, depending on the type of soap you are making.

You will mostly likely have glass bowls and a large metal spoon lying around in your kitchen that doesn't really get used. These are great and really needed for mixing the lye into the water. Metal or even plastic measuring cups are handy and so are measuring spoons. A rubber spatula is handy for scraping the last bit of soap out of the pot as you are pouring it into the mold; the soap does start setting rather quickly the longer it sits. If you do not have any extra (remember, you want to keep these separate from food equipment) many thrift stores will carry these items.

As you develop your talent, other items may be purchased to make designs in the soap.

There are several different basic ingredients you will need to make soap, including, but not limited to: base oils and fats, distilled or filtered water, lye, and any essential oils and colorants you may want to add. Each oil, fat, essential oils, and colorants will bring a different property to the soap. Each recipe that you follow should be followed exactly until you understand how these work together.

I am not going to get into the different properties of each oil, etc. because there are plenty of resources already available on the subject. This small e-book is for introductory purposes only to get you the basic information about soap making; however, with that being said, I will go over the basics of these ingredients in a broad sense.

These three are the most basic ingredients needed to make soap:

Base oils are used in each and every recipe. There will be a certain weight needed for each oil, depending on what oil is being used for any given recipe. All oils have a different combination of vitamins, minerals, and fatty acids so it is imperative that the weight of each oil be used in the soap recipe exactly, otherwise, the hard bar you were intending to make came out too soft, for example. Usually, each soap recipe will have at least different three different types of oils in it. Coconut oil, olive oil, grapeseed oil, avocado oil, shea butter, and cocoa butter are just a few of the different oils that can be used in your soaps.

Water is another major ingredient that is used in each and every recipe. This is what the lye gets mixed into to start the chemical process of soap. Water will also aid in how quickly the recipe will come to trace. I recommend distilled or filtered water bought from the store to ensure all purities from faucet water are non-existent.

Lye is the last of the major ingredients used for soap. Lye should always be poured into the water, not the other way around. Many stores do not carry 100% lye anymore, so an online retailer is usually the best way to go. I usually buy my lye from Amazon and this is a good deal for 6 lbs. of lye:

https://www.amazon.com/gp/product/B008XN4POI/ref=as_li_tl?ie=UTF8&camp=1789&creative=9325&creativeASIN=B008XN4POI&linkCode=as2&tag=simplyagritsl-20&linkId=5ab7lcc83c3c3505746e8d9f3d630f9f

at $35.99. Each of the recipes that are on my blog calls for lye; it is for the harder soap bars, not the liquid soap.

One word of note here: once you become familiar with the soap making process and have made a few batches, there are plenty of "lye calculators" online that can help ensure you use the right amount of oils, lye, and water to create your own soap. However, I have always found that to be confusing until I found this lye calculator. It gives clear step-by-step instructions so you will know exactly what amount to use of each ingredient to create your one-of-a-kind soap. And of course, I will definitely want to try it too!!

Extra ingredients that are nice to have, but not necessary are the essential oils, colorants, herbs, spices, dried flowers, oats, coffee grounds, and different milks. This list could be endless. These will make your soaps smell good and look amazing.

Essential oils help add amazing smells to your soaps. There are hundreds of different essential oils out on the market; however, you do not need to stock up on every scent. Just get the scents that matter to you most in the beginning.

Colorants add color to your soap; there are plenty of resources that can add color to your soaps, including any herbs or spices that you use. You are wanting to make sure you use all natural, make sure you use herbs, spices, coffee grounds, or clays that will color your soap. Here at Amazon, is mica powder that can be used for colorants. This is a natural additive.

Herbs, spices, and dried flowers not only can add color, but also can add other benefits for your soaps; appealing and exfoliation are just but a couple. The options are endless.

Oats, coffee grounds, milks, and even honey are wonderful to use in soaps. I have one bar that uses oats, goat milk, cinnamon and honey! It is a lovely bar.

Chapter Three: The Actual Process of Soap Making

In this chapter, I will show you the cold-process soap making method as this is the process I learned with and truly love since you control all the ingredients.

Cold-Process Soap Making

What is meant by cold-process? This means that the soap is made without using heat. The only heat used if for melting down the oils to use. The actual soap batter is closer to that of room temperature. The ideal temperature I use when making soap is around 100° F once it cools. I like using the cold-process because not only do you control all the ingredients being put into the soap, but you also have much more control over the beauty of the soap, like adding swirls, dried flowers, etc.

1) Always make sure you gather all your ingredients, down to the last spice. Nothing is worse than when you start to make a batch of soap, knowing you have that one ingredient and when you go to fetch it, low-and-behold, it isn't there. So ensure you have all your ingredients first. Then gather all your supplies needed, including your safety gear for working with lye.

2) After you have gathered all your ingredients and supplies, you will then weigh all your ingredients: the oils, water, lye, essential oils, and any other additives you are using. Using a digital kitchen scale that can go by ounces is what I recommend using. Start with the oils and then combine them all into your large stock pot. Then measure your water in a large glass bowl and then measure your lye in a separate container (you can even use a Ziploc type bag, if needed). The lye must be poured into the water; not the other way around.

3) Heat the oils over medium-low heat until fully dissolved. Make sure you are wearing your safety gear and then mix the lye into the water, stirring with a large metal spoon until completely dissolved; this is usually only a few seconds.

4) Once both the oils have melted and the lye/water has been mixed, these will need to cool. Most recipes will have them cool between 100° F - 110° F. Some recipes may need to temperature to be slightly cooler, just make sure you always read through the recipe first to know exactly what to expect with each one.
If they do not cool at the same time, you can use a cold-water bath or a hot-water bath to get the temperature where it needs to be. Just fill your sink with either the cold water or hot water and set the oils or lye/water into the sink of water until the desired temperature is reached.

5) Once both have reached the right temperature, carefully pour the lye/water mixture into the oils and then with your stick blender, mix for

about 2 minutes, and then let the mixture rest for about 5 minutes. Continue doing this until your soap mixture comes to light trace. You will know once you reach light trace when you can create a trail on the top of the mixture by drizzling it over.

6) Once the mixture is at light trace, then add any additives the recipe calls for and continue mixing again for another 30 seconds to 1 minute. Powered colorants are usually mixed with 1 cup of water ahead of time and then blended in at this step to prevent lumps or saved until after the mixture is poured into soap molds for a finishing touch.

7) After the mixing is completed, you will pour the mixture into your mold and make any designs at this stage, if using. Cover with parchment paper. Insulate the mold, if required, for at least 24 hours, with a blanket. Check your soap after 24 hours, and if still too soft, wait another 12-24 hours.

8) After you are able to remove the soap from the mold, cut into bars and let it

cure in a ventilated area for 4-6 weeks.

9) Your soaps are ready to use!! Congratulations!!!

Glossary:

Cold-Process: the making of soap at room temperature. The only heat used is during the melting phase of the oils. This process makes a nice hard bar.

Curing: the process of letting the soap harden for 4 to 6 weeks. Soap can be used immediately after a few days, however, letting it cure allows the soap to harden fully, excess water evaporating, and will last longer in the shower.

Fatty Acids: a carboxylic acid consisting of a hydrocarbon chain and a terminal carboxyl group, especially any of those occurring as esters in fats and oils.

Some of the more popular fatty acids:
- Lauric Acid: Hard bar, excellent cleansing, lots of fluffy lather; can be drying to skin.
- Linoleic Acid: Conditioning, silky feel
- Myristic acid: Hard bar, cleansing, fluffy lather
- Oleic acid: Conditioning, slippery feel, stingy lather, kind to skin
- Palmitic acid: Hard bar, cleansing, stable lather

> ➢ Ricinoleic acid: Softer bar, conditioning, moisturizing, lots of fluffy stable lather, kind to skin
> ➢ Stearic acid: Hard, long lasting bar, stable lather

Gel Phase: soap gets as hot as 180°F and develops a gelatinous appearance, this is not required; more of a personal preference. It does not affect the usage of the bar.

Hot-Process: the making of soap by heating it over low heat. It is ready to use immediately after it cools, but it does have a different texture that the cold-process method.

Saponification Value: a measure of the total free and combined acids especially in fats and oils expressed as the number of milligrams of potassium hydroxide required for the complete SAPONIFICATION of one gram of substance.

Saponification: this is the chemical reaction of the lye/water mixing with the oils when combined to produce a glycerol molecule and a fatty acid salt, called soap.

Soap Ash: this is an uneven, white, ashy film on soap. This can form when unsaponified lye reacts with naturally-occurring carbon dioxide in the air. It does not harm the soap or make it unusable; it just isn't as eye-appealing.

Sodium Hydroxide (NaOH): this is the chemical name for lye, which is an alkali, and it is mixed with water then added to the oils to make a hard soap. Potassium Hydroxide (KOH) is used to make a liquid soap.

Trace: the phase when the soap is ready to pour; this can be at a light trace, medium trace, or thick trace. Dribble some over the top of the mixture to know where your trace is currently when mixing.

Castile Soap

This is a basic soap recipe that has a good lather; also able to use a variety of different scents to make this unique.

Materials:

- 25 ounces of virgin olive oil
- 7 ounces of coconut oil
- 4 ounces of lye
- 12 ounces water (distilled or filtered is best)
- 1 ounce of your favorite 100% pure essential oil.

Instructions:

1. Heat the oils in a large pot over medium-low heat until they are melted. Remove from heat and let cool to between 100° F to 110° F.
2. Mix the lye into the water while the oils are heating. Carefully add the lye to the water and stir with a metal spoon until completely dissolved. Allow to cool to between 100° F to 110° F. You

can use a hot- or cold-water bath to adjust the temperatures as necessary to allow both the oils and lye water to reach the same approximate temperature at the same time.

3. While both the oils and lye water are cooling, prepare your molds. Line a mold with parchment paper, if needed, to be able to contain the full amount of the soap, approximately 3 pounds.

4. Combine the oils and lye water and bring to trace by using a stick mixer and mix for approximately 2-3 minutes and let rest for about 5 minutes. Continue this process until the mixture is at a light trace.

5. Add the essential oil of your choice and mix for other 30 seconds to one minute.

6. Pour the mixture into the mold and cover with parchment paper and insulate for at least 24 hours.

7. Cut and cure the soap for about 4 weeks. If the mixture seems really soft when removing the soap from the mold or cutting the soap, rewrap in blanket for another 24 hours and then cut into bars and let cure for the 4 weeks.

Basic 3-Oil Soap

Materials:

- 9.4 ounces of vegetable shortening
- 6 ounces of olive oil
- 6 ounces of coconut oil
- 3 ounces of lye
- 7 ounces of distilled water
- 1 ounce of any essential oil of your choice

Instructions:

1. Carefully add the lye to the water, ensuring you are wearing your safety gear. While this cools, heat all the oils until completely melted.
2. Let both the lye/water mixture and the oils cool to 100° F - 110° F.
3. Add the lye/water mixture to the oils and using the stick blender, blend for about 2 minutes and let rest for about 5 minutes. Continue this until it reaches a light trace and then add the essential oil.
4. Continue mixing off and on until light/medium trace.

5. Pour the mixture into the mold, insulate, and let it set for 36 to 48 hours. Once soap is easily removed from mold, unmold it. If not, continue to let it set for another 12 hours.
6. Unmold, cut, and let the soaps cure for 4 to 6 weeks.

Aloe Vera Soap

Materials:

- 14.9 ounces of coconut oil
- 13.4 ounces of olive oil
- 2.5 ounces of Shea butter
- 10.5 ounces of lard
- 6.7 ounces of lye
- 9.9 ounces of distilled water
- 9.6 ounces of aloe gel and water combined
- 1 ounce of any essential oil of your choice

Instructions:

1. Carefully add the lye to the water, ensuring you are wearing your safety gear. While this cools, heat all the oils until completely melted.
2. Let both the lye/water mixture and the oils cool to 100° F - 110° F.
3. Add the lye/water mixture to the oils and using the stick blender, blend for about 2 minutes and let rest for about 5 minutes. Continue this until just before a trace appears and then add the aloe gel and essential oil.

4. Continue mixing off and on until light/medium trace.
5. Pour the mixture into the mold, cover and insulate, and let it set for 24 to 48 hours. Once soap is easily removed from mold, unmold it. If not, continue to let it set for another 12 hours.
6. Unmold, cut, and let the soaps cure for 4 to 6 weeks.

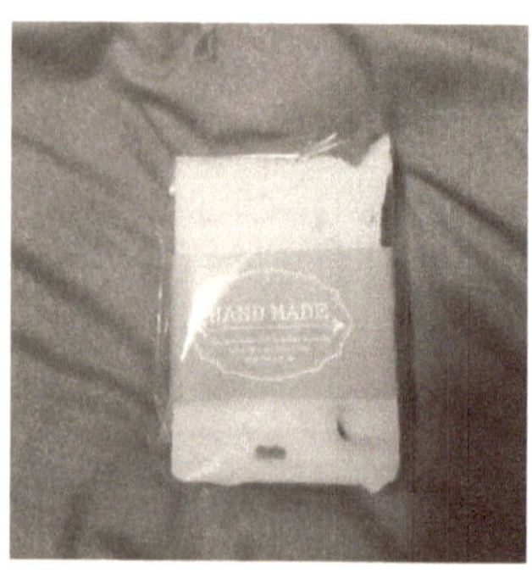

Cinnamon, Oats, & Honey Soap

Materials:

- 8 ounces of coconut oil
- 9 ounces of olive oil
- 8 ounces of lard
- 5 ounces of castor oil
- 3 ounces of grapeseed oil
- 4 ounces of lye
- 8 ounces of distilled water
- 4 ounces of goat milk
- ½ cup ground oats
- 1 ounce cinnamon leaf essential oil
- 1 tablespoon raw honey, preferably with the honeycomb

Instructions:

1. Combine the water and goat milk 1 to 2 hours in advance and set in freezer until a slush forms; do NOT let if freeze.
2. Process the oats by grinding them, either by hand or a blender until they are in a fine powder.
3. Add the lye into the milk/water mixture ¼ amount at a time; let cool for about 15 minutes and repeat

process until all the lye is mixed in. If you add all the lye too quickly, you could burn the milk/water and it will be more of a dark brown bar.

4. As the lye and milk/water mixture are cooling, mix all the oils together and heat over medium low heat until all have melted.
5. Let both the lye/milk/water mixture and the oils cool to 90° F - 100° F.
6. Prepare your mold while they are cooling; line with parchment paper, if needed.
7. Add the lye/water mixture to the oils and using the stick blender, blend for about 2 minutes and let rest for about 5 minutes. Continue this until just before a trace appears and then add the cinnamon leaf essential oil, oats, and honey and blend another 30 seconds.
8. Pour into mold, cover with parchment paper (do not insulate), and let it set for 24 hours. Once soap is easily removed from mold, unmold it. If not, continue to let it set for another 12 hours.
9. Unmold, cut, and let the soaps cure for 4 to 6 weeks.

Cinnamon Soap

Materials:

- 20 ounces of olive oil
- 9 ounces of coconut oil
- 3 ounces of hazelnut oil
- 2 ounces of castor oil
- 4.8 ounces of lye
- 12.9 ounces of distilled water
- 1 ounce cinnamon essential oil
- 1 tablespoon ground cinnamon

Instructions:

1.	Combine all the oils and heat over medium-low heat until they are melted. Let cool until around 90° F - 100° F.
2.	Add the lye into the water mixture and let cool to around 90° F - 100° F.
3.	Prepare your mold while they are cooling; line with parchment paper, if needed.
4.	Add the lye/water mixture to the oils and using the stick blender, blend for about 2 minutes and let rest for about 5 minutes. Continue this until a light trace appears and then add

the cinnamon essential oil and blend another 30 seconds.

5. Separate one cup of the soap mixture and add in the ground cinnamon and whisk until well-blended and there are no lumps.
6. Pour the rest of the soap mixture into the mold, and then carefully pour the separated mixture over the mold, back and forth across the length of the mold. Using a rubber spatula, make designs with the darker cinnamon mixture dipping the spatula down into the mixture and moving it up and down.
7. Cover with parchment paper and insulate, and let it set for 24 hours. Once soap is easily removed from mold, unmold it. If not, continue to let it set for another 12 hours.
8. Unmold, cut, and let the soaps cure for 4 to 6 weeks.

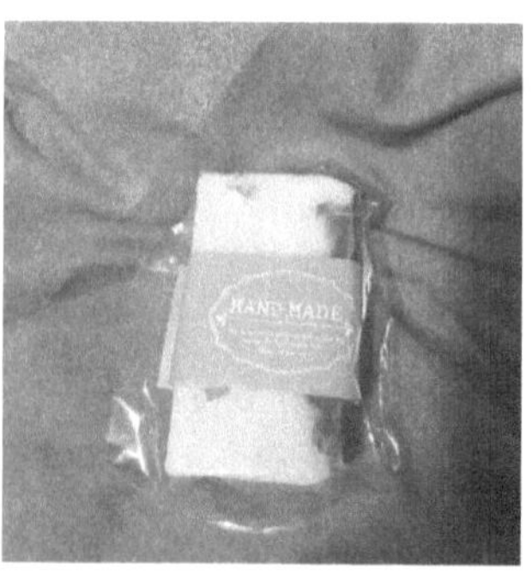

Peppermint and Basil Soap

Materials:

- 12 ounces of lard
- 9 ounces of coconut oil
- 4 ounces of olive oil
- 3 ounces of grapeseed oil
- 3 ounces of castor oil
- 2 ounces of cocoa butter
- 4.3 ounces of lye
- 12.9 ounces of distilled water
- 0.5 ounce peppermint essential oil
- 0.5 ounce basil essential oil
- 1 Tbsp dried peppermint flakes

Instructions:

1. Combine all the oils and heat over medium-low heat until they are melted. Let cool until around 100° F - 110° F.
2. Add the lye into the water mixture and let cool to around 100° F - 110° F.
3. Prepare your mold while they are cooling; line with parchment paper, if needed.
4. Add the lye/water mixture to the oils and using the stick blender,

blend for about 2 minutes and let rest for about 5 minutes. Continue this until a light trace appears and then add the peppermint and basil essential oils and blend another 30 seconds.

5.   Pour the soap mixture into the mold, and then sprinkle the peppermint flakes on top.
6.   Cover with parchment paper and insulate, and let it set for 24 hours. Once soap is easily removed from mold, unmold it. If not, continue to let it set for another 12 hours.
7.   Unmold, cut, and let the soaps cure for 4 to 6 weeks.

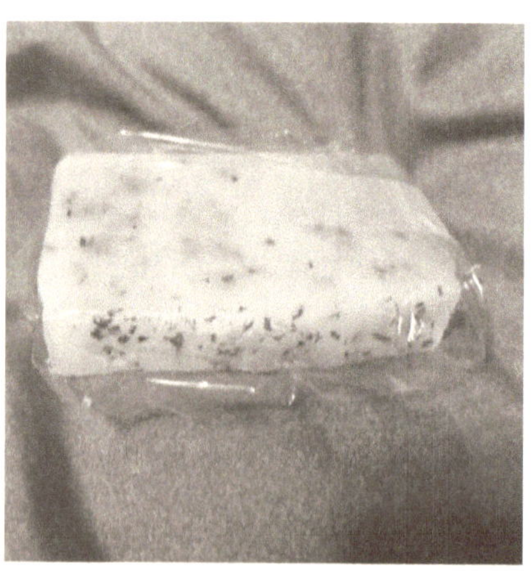

Mineral & Dead Sea Salt Soap

Materials:

- 27 ounces of coconut oil
- 2 ounces of olive oil
- 1 ounce of castor oil
- 4.3 ounces of lye
- 4 ounces of goat milk
- 7.4 ounces of distilled water
- 1 ounce of your favorite essential oil
- 30 ounces of mineral and dead sea salt

Instructions:

1. Combine the water and goat milk 1 to 2 hours in advance and set in freezer until a slush forms; do NOT let if freeze.
2. Add the lye into the milk/water mixture ¼ amount at a time; let cool for about 15 minutes and repeat process until all the lye is mixed in. If you add all the lye too quickly, you could burn the milk/water and it will be more of a dark brown bar. Let cool to around 90° F - 100° F.

3.   While the lye mixture cools, combine all the oils and heat over medium-low heat until they are melted. Let cool until around 90° F - 100° F.
4.   Prepare your mold while they are cooling; line with parchment paper, if needed.
5.   Add the lye & milk/water mixture to the oils and using the stick blender, blend for about 2 minutes and let rest for about 5 minutes. Continue this until a light trace appears and then add the essential oil and salt and blend another 30 seconds.
6.   Pour the soap mixture into the mold. Cover with parchment paper and let it set for about 3-4 hours. Do not let it set too long.
7.   Unmold, cut, and let the soaps cure for 2 to 3 weeks.
8.   Soaps with salt do not take as long to set or cure, BE CAREFUL!!

Allergy Help Soap

Materials:

- 10 ounces of olive oil
- 9 ounces of coconut oil
- 4 ounces of sweet almond oil
- 4 ounces of cocoa butter
- 3 ounces of shea butter
- 4.1 ounces of lye
- 12.5 ounces of distilled water
- 0.35 ounce peppermint essential oil
- 0.35 ounce lavender essential oil
- 0.35 ounce lemon essential oil

Instructions:

1. Combine all the oils and heat over medium-low heat until they are melted. Let cool until around 100° F - 110° F.
2. Add the lye into the water mixture and let cool to around 100° F - 110° F.
3. Prepare your mold while they are cooling; line with parchment paper, if needed.
4. Add the lye/water mixture to the oils and using the stick blender, blend for about 2 minutes and let rest

for about 5 minutes. Continue this until a light trace appears and then add the essential oils and blend another 30 seconds.
5.	Pour the soap mixture into the mold, and cover with parchment paper and insulate, and let it set for 24 hours. Once soap is easily removed from mold, unmold it. If not, continue to let it set for another 12 hours.
6.	Unmold, cut, and let the soaps cure for 4 to 6 weeks.

Lavender Soap

Materials:

- 9 ounces of olive oil
- 9 ounces of lard
- 7 ounces of coconut oil
- 3 ounces of castor oil
- 2 ounces of hazelnut oil
- 2 ounces of cocoa butter
- 1 ounce of shea butter
- 4.6 ounces of lye
- 12.5 ounces of distilled water
- 1 ounce of lavender essential oil
- 1 Tbsp. dried alkanet root powder
- 1 -2 Tbsp. dried lavender

Instructions:

1. Combine all the oils and heat over medium-low heat until they are melted. Let cool until around 100° F - 110° F.
2. Add the lye into the water mixture and let cool to around 100° F - 110° F.
3. Prepare your mold while they are cooling; line with parchment paper, if needed.

4. Add the lye/water mixture to the oils and using the stick blender, blend for about 2 minutes and let rest for about 5 minutes. Continue this until a light trace appears and then add the lavender essential oil and blend another 30 seconds.
5. Transfer 1 cup of the soap mixture to a separate bowl and mix in the alkanet root powder and whisk until well blended and there are no lumps.
6. Pour the rest of the soap mixture into the mold; slowly pour the alkanet root soap mixture over the mold and then using the whisk, make swirly marks into the top layer. Sprinkle the dried lavender on top.
7. Cover with parchment paper and insulate, and let it set for 24 hours. Once soap is easily removed from mold, unmold it. If not, continue to let it set for another 12 hours.
8. Unmold, cut, and let the soaps cure for 4 to 6 weeks.